The New Mediterranean Diet Cookbook

Quick And Easy Mediterranean Meals For Busy People

Ben Cooper

© **Copyright 2020 - All rights reserved.**

The content contained within this book may not be reproduced, duplicated or transmitted without direct written permission from the author or the publisher.
Under no circumstances will any blame or legal responsibility be held against the publisher, or author, for any damages, reparation, or monetary loss due to the information contained within this book. Either directly or indirectly.

Legal Notice:
This book is copyright protected. This book is only for personal use. You cannot amend, distribute, sell, use, quote or paraphrase any part, or the content within this book, without the consent of the author or publisher.

Disclaimer Notice:
Please note the information contained within this document is for educational and entertainment purposes only. All effort has been executed to present accurate, up to date, and reliable, complete information. No warranties of any kind are declared or implied. Readers acknowledge that the author is not engaging in the rendering of legal, financial, medical or professional advice. The content within this book has been derived from various sources. Please consult a licensed professional before attempting any techniques outlined in this book.

By reading this document, the reader agrees that under no circumstances is the author responsible for any losses, direct or indirect, which are incurred as a result of the use of information contained within this document, including, but not limited to, — errors, omissions, or inaccuracies.

Table of contents

Roasted brussels sprouts with turmeric and mustard seeds.................. 7
Avocado egg boats 9
Stuffed Mushrooms 11
Kale with Pine Nuts 12
Buckwheat Tuna Casserole 15
Scallops with Mushrooms 17
Courgette Risotto 19
Braised Leek with Pine Nuts 21
Parsley Butter Shrimp 23
Foil Baked Salmon 25
Baked Zesty Tilapia 27
Prawns with Asparagus 29
Tuna and Kale 31
Minty Soup 33
Sweet and Gorgeus Lentil Stew 37
Delicious Meatball Soup for the Spanish 37
Rice Rolls Preparation 39
Rice Stew with Squid 41
Creamy Millet 43
Oatmeal Cakes 45
Yogurt Buckwheat 47
Halloumi Buckwheat Bowl 49
Aromatic Green Millet 51
Quinoa with Pumpkin 53
Almond Quinoa 55
Mushroom Quinoa Skillet 59

Strawberry Quinoa Bowl	59
Stir-Fried Farro	63
Quick Farro Skillet	63
Bulgur Bowl	65
Boiled Bulgur with Kale	67
Chicken and Rice Soup	69
Tomato Bulgur	71
Well spiced Lentil Soup with sour taste	73
Delicious and entertaining Lamb Veggie Soup	75
Bulgur Mix	77
Aromatic Baked Brown Rice	79
Aromatic Barley Pilaf	81
Basmati Rice Pilaf Mix	83
Brown Rice Salad with Asparagus, Goat Cheese, and Lemon	85
Carrot-Almond-Bulgur Salad	87
Chickpea-Spinach Bulgur	89
Classic Baked Brown Rice	91
Classic Italian Seafood Risotto	93
Classic Stovetop White Rice	95
Chicken Sausage Minestrone	97
Italian Lentil soup	99
Smoked chicken sausage soup	101
Lemon Chicken Soup	103
Tuscan Vegetable Pasta Soup	105
Dairy Free Zucchini Soup	107
Farro Stew with Kale & Cannellini Beans	109

Roasted brussels sprouts with turmeric and mustard seeds

Preparation Time: 30 minutes
Cooking Time: 20 minutes
Servings: 2

Ingredients:

1 teaspoon oil
1/2 teaspoon (0.5 tsp) black mustard seeds
1/4 teaspoon (0.25 tsp) turmeric
Cloves of garlic finely chopped teaspoon or more sesame seeds
Cups (176 g) Brussels sprouts
1/2 teaspoon (0.5 tsp) coriander powder
1 green chili finely chopped
1/2 teaspoon (0.5 tsp) cumin seeds
1/2 teaspoon (0.5 tsp) garam masala optional cayenne to taste
1/2 teaspoon (0.5 tsp) salt or to taste
1/4 cup (62.5 ml) water
cilantro and lemon for garnish

Directions:

1. Heat oil in a large skillet. When hot, put cumin and mustard seeds and cook until they change color or start to pop. Further, put curry leaves, garlic and chili carefully. Cook for a minute.

2. Now, add Brussels sprouts. Cook for 5 minutes until some edges get golden brown. Stir when needed.

3.Put sesame seeds, mix in and cook for a minute. Mix in ground spices, salt and mix in and cook for a minute.

4.Add water. Cover and cook for 7 to 9 minute to steam the sprouts.

5.Finely, adjust salt. Add a some lemon and cilantro and serve.

Avocado egg boats

Preparation Time: 40min
Cooking Time: 8 minutes
Servings: 4

Ingredients:

Freshly ground black pepper
Ripe avocados, halved and pitted slices bacon
large eggs Kosher salt
Freshly chopped chives, for garnish

Directions:

1. Firstly, preheat oven to 350°. Scoop about 1 tbsp. worth of avocado out of each half;

2. Put hollowed avocados in a baking dish, then crack eggs into a bowl, one at a time. Use a spoon, transfer one yolk to each avocado half, and then spoon in as much egg white as you can fit.

3. Add in salt and pepper and bake until whites are set and yolks are no longer runny, 20 to 25 minutes. (Cover with foil if avocados are beginning to brown.)

4. In the meantime, in a large skillet over medium heat, cook bacon until crisp, 8 minutes, and then transfer to a paper towel-lined plate and chop.

5. Finally, top avocados with bacon and chives before serving.

Stuffed Mushrooms

Preparation Time: 10 minutes
Cooking Time: 20 minutes
Servings: 3

Ingredients:

20 large mushrooms, washed
1 tbsp. extra virgin olive oil
1 cup broccoli, chopped
1 medium red onion, diced
1 tsp garlic, minced
¼ cup capers
½ tsp. Dried oregano
½ tsp. dried parsley tbsp. feta cheese
1 tbsp. breadcrumbs Salt and pepper to taste

Directions:

1. Preheat oven to 425 ° F.

2. Remove the stems from the mushrooms carefully and dice them.

3. Place mushroom tops in a single layer on a baking sheet, with the hole facing up, and bake for 5 minutes.

4. Put olive oil in a pan with the diced mushrooms stems, broccoli, onion, garlic, capers, oregano, parsley and salt, and pepper.

5. Cook for 7 minutes. Add feta and breadcrumbs.

6. Stuff mushrooms with mixture and bake for 8 minutes.

Kale with Pine Nuts

Preparation Time: 10minutes
Cooking Time: 10 minutes
Servings: 4

Ingredients:

1 tbsp. olive oil garlic cloves, minced
1½ lb. fresh kale, tough ribs removed and chopped
¼ cup water
1 tsp. red wine vinegar
Salt and add black pepper, to taste
1 tbsp. pine nuts

Directions:

1. Heat the olive oil in a large wok over medium heat and sauté the garlic for about 1 minute.

2. Add the kale and cook for 4 minutes.

3. Add the water, vinegar, salt, and black pepper and cook for 5 minutes.

4. Remove from heat and stir in the pine nuts.

5. Serve immediately.

Buckwheat Tuna Casserole

Preparation Time: 10 minutes
Cooking Time: 35 minutes
Servings: 2

Ingredients:

Tbsp. butter
10- oz. package buckwheat ramen noodles
Cups boiling water
1/3 cup dry red wine
Cups of milk
Tbsp. dried parsley
Tsp. Turmeric
½ tsp. curry powder
Tbsp. all-Purpose flour cups celery, chopped
1 cup frozen peas
Cans tuna, drained

Directions:

1. Grease your pot with butter.

2. Place buckwheat ramen noodles in a large bowl and pour boiling water to cover.

3. Let it sit for 7 minutes, or until noodles separate when prodded with a fork.

4. In a separate bowl, whisk together red wine, milk, parsley, turmeric, and flour.

5. Fold in celery, peas, and tuna.

6. Drain the ramen and place it into the crockpot, pouring the tuna mixture over the top.

7. Mix to combine.

8. Cover and cook for an hour, stirring occasionally.

Scallops with Mushrooms

Preparation Time: 5 minutes
Cooking Time: 10 minutes
Servings: 4

Ingredients:
1 lb. scallops
Tbsp. olive oil
Scallions, chopped
½ cup mushrooms, sliced
Tbsp. almonds, chopped
1 cup coconut cream

Directions:

1. Heat a pan with the oil over medium heat; add the scallions and the mushrooms and sauté for 2 minutes.

2. Add the scallops cook over medium heat for 8 minutes more, divide into bowls and serve.

Courgette Risotto

Preparation Time: 10 minutes
Cooking Time: 8 minutes
Servings: 8

Ingredients:

Tbsp. olive oil
Cloves garlic, finely chopped
lb. Arborio rice
Tomatoes, chopped
Tsp. chopped rosemary
Courgettes, finely diced
1 ¼ cups peas, fresh or frozen
1cups hot vegetable stock chopped
Salt and ground black pepper to taste

Directions:

1. Place a large, heavy-bottomed pan over medium heat. Add oil.

2. When the oil is heated, add onion and sauté until translucent.

3. Stir in the tomatoes and cook until soft. Next, stir in the rice and rosemary. Mix well. Add half the stock and cook until dry. Stir frequently.

4. Add remaining stock and cook for 3-4 minutes.

5. Add courgette and peas and cook until rice is tender.

6. Add salt and pepper to taste.

7.Stir in the basil and let it sit for 5 minutes.

8.Serve warm and enjoy

Braised Leek with Pine Nuts

Preparation Time: 45 minutes
Cooking Time: 15 minutes
Servings: 2

Ingredients:

Tbsp. Ghee tsp Olive oil pieces Leek
oz. Vegetable broth
A bunch of fresh parsley
1 tbsp. fresh oregano
1 tbsp. Pine nuts (roasted)

Directions:

1. Cut the leek into thin rings and finely chop the herbs.

2. Roast the pine nuts in a dry pan over medium heat.

3. Melt the ghee together with the olive oil in a large pan.

4. Cook the leek until golden brown for 5 minutes, stirring constantly.

5. Add the vegetable broth and cook for another 10 minutes until the leek is tender.

6. Stir in the herbs and sprinkle the pine nuts on the dish just before serving.

Parsley Butter Shrimp

Preparation Time: 10 minutes
Cooking Time: 22 minutes
Servings: 4

Ingredients:

1 lb. shrimp, peeled and deveined
Tbsp. butter, divided
Cloves garlic, minced
½ cup chicken stock
Tbsp. parsley, minced
Tbsp. Lemon juice
¼ tsp. Red pepper flakes
½ tsp. Black pepper
½ tsp. kosher salt

Directions:

1. Heat 2 tbsp. of butter in a large, heavy-bottomed skillet over medium heat.

2. Add the shrimp to the skillet and sprinkle with salt and pepper.

3. Cook, occasionally stirring, for 5 minutes or until shrimp is cooked through.

4. Remove shrimp to a plate and set aside.

5. Add the garlic to the skillet and cook, constantly stirring, for 30 seconds.

6. Add the chicken stock and whisk to combine. Simmer until the stock has reduced by half, about 7 minutes.

7. Add the remaining 4 tbsp. of butter, lemon juice, and red pepper to the sauce. Stir to melt the butter and cook for two more minutes.

8. Remove from heat and return the shrimp to the sauce. Sprinkle the parsley over the top and stir to combine.

9. Serve immediately.

Foil Baked Salmon

Preparation Time: 8 minutes
Cooking Time: 20 minutes
Servings: 2

Ingredients:

Salmon fillets
Asparagus spears
1 tsp. dried oregano
Slices onion
1 tsp. fresh parsley, chopped
Slices lemon
1 tbsp. extra virgin olive oil Salt and black pepper to taste

Directions:

1. Preheat oven to 400° F.

2. In a medium bowl, place the two pieces of salmon.

3. Pour 1 tbsp. Of olive oil and sprinkle salt, pepper, and dried oregano.

4. Cut two sheets of foil. It has to be big enough to wrap the salmon and asparagus. First place asparagus, about 8 spears, on the sheet of foil.

5. Layer fillets over asparagus, then top each with about two onion slices and two lemon slices.

6. Wrap sides of foil inward over salmon, fold on top and bottom of the foil to enclose.

7.Place foil packets in a single layer on a baking sheet.

8.Bake in preheated oven for about 15 minutes. Unwrap and using a large spatula, transfer the foil packets to plates. Serve warm!

Baked Zesty Tilapia

Preparation Time: 10 minutes
Cooking Time: 10 minutes
Servings: 4

Ingredients:

Tilapia fillets
¼ cup unsalted butter, melted
Cloves garlic, minced
Tbsp. freshly squeezed lemon juice to taste Zest of 1 lemon
tbsp. chopped fresh parsley leaves Kosher
Salt and black pepper to taste

Directions:

1. Preheat the oven to 425° F.

2. Lightly grease a baking dish or coat with non-stick spray.

3. In a small bowl, whisk together butter, lemon juice, garlic, and lemon zest and set aside.

4. Season the fillets with salt and pepper, taste and place onto the prepared baking dish and drizzle with butter mixture.

5. Place into the oven and bake until fish flakes easily with a fork, about 10 minutes.

6. Serve immediately, garnished with parsley.

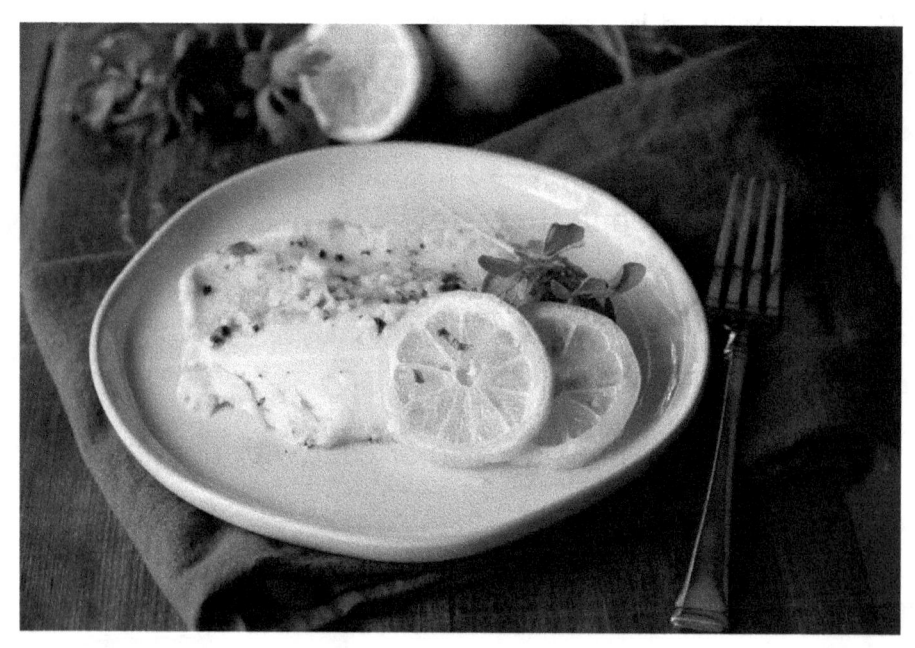

Prawns with Asparagus

Preparation Time: 10 minutes
Cooking Time: 12 minutes
Servings: 4

Ingredients:

Tbsp. olive oil
1 lb. prawns, peeled, and deveined
1 lb. asparagus, trimmed
Salt and black pepper, to taste
1 tsp. garlic, minced
1 tsp. fresh ginger, minced
1 tbsp. low-sodium soy sauce
Tbsp. lemon juice

Directions:

1. In a wok, heat 2 tbsp. of oil over medium-high heat and cook the prawns with salt and black pepper for about 4 minutes.

2. With a slotted spoon, transfer the prawns into a bowl and set aside.

3. In the same wok, heat remaining 1 tbsp. Of oil over medium-high heat and cook the asparagus, ginger, garlic, salt, and black pepper and sauté for about 7 minutes, stirring frequently.

4. Stir in the prawns and soy sauce and cook for about 1 minute.

5. Stir in the lemon juice and remove from the heat.

6.Serve hot.

Tuna and Kale

Preparation Time: 5 minutes
Cooking Time: 20 minutes
Servings: 4

Ingredients:

1 lb. tuna fillets, boneless, skinless and cubed
Tbsp. olive oil
1 cup kale, torn
½ cup cherry tomatoes, cubed
1 yellow onion, chopped

Directions:

1. Heat a pan with the oil over medium heat.

2. Add the onion and sauté for 5 minutes.

3. Add the tuna and the other ingredients.

4. Toss and cook everything for 15 minutes more, divide between plates and serve.

Minty Soup

Preparation and cooking: 35 minutes.
Serves: 6

Ingredients:

2 chopped garlic cloves
1 cup water
2 tbsp olive oil
¼ cup heavy cream
2 cups vegetable stock
2 chopped shallots
1 tbsp lemon juice
4 chopped mint leaves
½ tsp dried oregano
Pepper and salt to taste
1 pound green peas

Directions:

1. In garlic and shallots, stir heated oil in a soup pot and cook until it's softened for 2 minutes.

2. then add oregano, green peas, stock, mint and water.

3. Cook for 15 minutes on a low heat after adding pepper and salt to taste.

4. In the lemon juice, stir and cook it for 2 more minutes.

5. Remove from heat when it is done and stir it in the cream.

6.Use an immersion blender to puree the soup immersion blender until it is smooth and creamy.

7.Best served chilled or warm.

Sweet and gorgeous Lentil Stew

Cooking and preparation: 45 minutes
Serves: 8

Ingredients:

3 cups water
1 can crushed tomatoes
2 tbsp extra virgin olive oil
2 chopped garlic cloves
2 diced carrots
2 cored and diced red bell peppers
1 diced celery stalk
½ tsp cumin seeds
½ tsp mustard seeds
2 chopped shallots
3 cups vegetable stock
Pepper and salt to taste
1 cup green lentils
Yogurt for serving

Directions:

1.In a soup pot, heat the oil and stir in the garlic and shallots. Add other Ingredients: after cooking it for 2 minutes.

2.On low heat, adjust the taste with pepper and salt for 30 minutes.

3.Top it with freshly chopped parsley or plain yogurt after serving the soup fresh and warm.

Delicious Meatball Soup for the Spanish

Cooking and preparation: 1 hour
Serves: 8

Ingredients:

6 cups water
1 can crushed tomatoes
1 egg
2 tbsp olive oil
1 diced celery stalk
1 chopped onion
2 cored and diced red bell peppers
2 cups vegetable stock
2 diced carrots
1 pound ground veal
2 tbsp chopped parsley
2 chopped garlic cloves
Pepper and salt to taste

Directions:

1.In a soup pot, heat the oil and stir in the garlic, stock, bell peppers, onions, carrots, water and celery. Bring to a boiling after seasoning with pepper and salt.

2.In a bowl, mix egg, veal and parsley in the meantime. Then boil them in boiling liquid after forming small meatballs.

3.Adjust the taste with pepper and salt after adding the tomatoes.

4.For 20 minutes, cook on very low heat.

5.Best served fresh and warm.

Rice Rolls Preparation

Time: 15 minutes
Cooking Time: 35 minutes
Servings: 6

Ingredients:

4 white cabbage leaves 4 oz ground chicken
½ tsp. garlic powder
¼ cup of long grain rice, cooked
½ cup chicken stock
½ cup tomatoes, chopped

Directions:

1. In the bowl, mix ground chicken, garlic powder, and rice.

2. Then put the rice mixture on every cabbage leaf and roll.

3. Arrange the rice rolls in the saucepan.

4. Add chicken stock and tomatoes and close the lid.

5. Cook the rice rolls for 35 minutes on low heat.

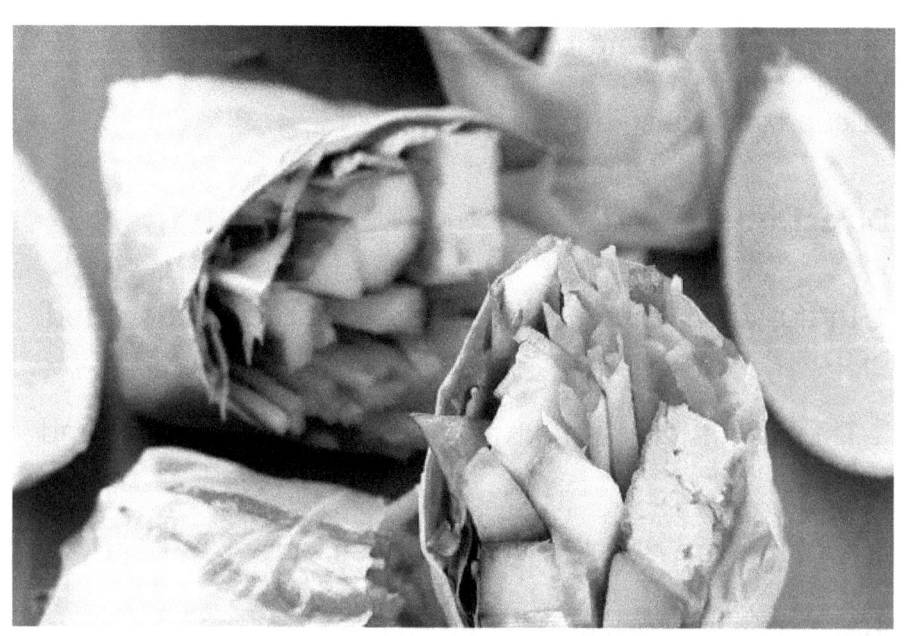

Rice Stew with Squid

Preparation Time: 10 minutes
Cooking Time: 30 minutes
Servings: 6

Ingredients:

5 oz long grain rice 4 oz squid, sliced
1 jalapeno pepper, chopped
½ cup tomatoes, chopped
1 onion, diced
2 cups chicken stock
1 tbsp. avocado oil

Directions:

1. Roast the onion with avocado oil in the skillet for 3-4 minutes or until the onion is light brown.

2. Add squid, jalapeno pepper, and tomatoes.

3. Cook the ingredients for 7 minutes.

4. Then cook rice with water for 15 minutes.

5. Add cooked rice in the squid mixture, stir, and cook for 3 minutes more.

Creamy Millet

Preparation Time: 10 minutes
Cooking Time: 10 minutes
Servings: 6

Ingredients:

½ cup millet
1 oz cream cheese
¼ tsp. salt
1.5 cup hot water

Directions:
1. Mix hot water and millet in the saucepan.

2. Boil it for 8 minutes on low heat

3. Add cream cheese and salt.

4. Carefully stir the cooked millet.

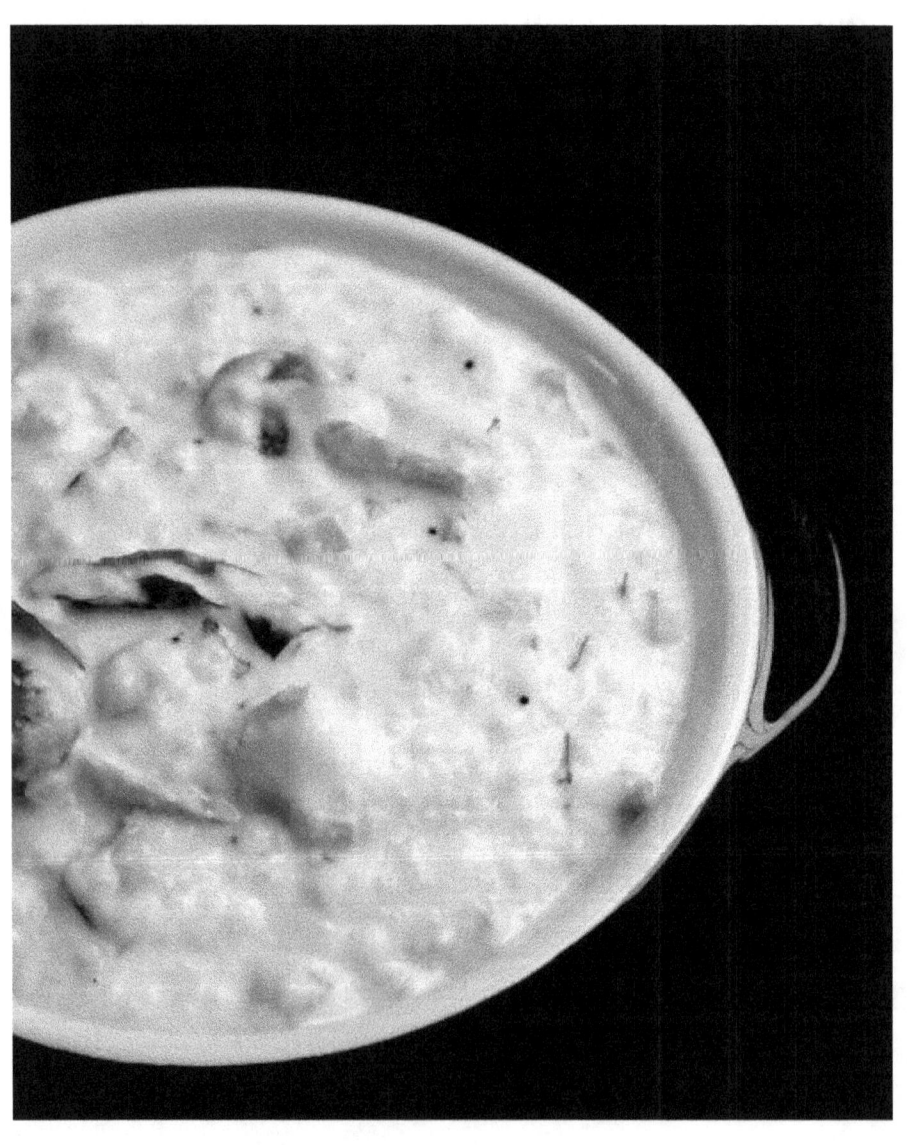

Oatmeal Cakes

Preparation Time: 15 minutes
Cooking Time: 7 minutes
Servings: 4

Ingredients:

½ cup oatmeal 1 egg, beaten
1 carrot, grated 1 tbsp.
olive oil 1 tsp. flax meal

Directions:

1. Put oatmeal, egg, grated carrot, and flax meal in the blender. Blend the mixture well.

2. Then heat olive oil in the skillet.

3. Make the medium-sized cakes from the oatmeal mixture and cook for 3 minutes per side on medium heat.

Yogurt Buckwheat

Preparation Time: 5 minutes
Cooking Time: 13 minutes
Servings: 2

Ingredients:

½ cup buckwheat
1.5 cup chicken stock
1 tbsp. plain yogurt

Directions:

1. Put all ingredients in the saucepan and close the lid.

2. Cook the meal for 13 minutes on low heat or until the buckwheat soaks all liquid

3. Carefully stir the cooked meal.

Halloumi Buckwheat Bowl

Preparation Time: 10 minutes

Cooking Time: 15 minutes

Servings: 4

Ingredients:
1 cup buckwheat cups chicken stock
4 oz halloumi cheese
1 tbsp. olive oil
½ tsp. dried thyme

Directions:
1. Mix chicken stock and buckwheat in the saucepan, boil, and cook for 7 minutes on medium heat.

2. After this, sprinkle the halloumi cheese with olive oil and dried thyme.

3. Grill it for 2 minutes per side or until the cheese is light brown.

4. Then put the cooked buckwheat in the bowls.

5. Chop the cheese roughly and top the buckwheat with it.

Aromatic Green Millet

Preparation Time: 10 minutes
Cooking Time: 7 minutes
Servings: 5

Ingredients:

1 cup millet
2 cups of water
4 tbsp. pesto sauce
¼ tsp. cayenne pepper

Directions:

1. Mix water and millet in the saucepan and boil for 7 minutes.

2. Then add cayenne pepper and pesto sauce.

3. Stir the millet until homogenous and green.

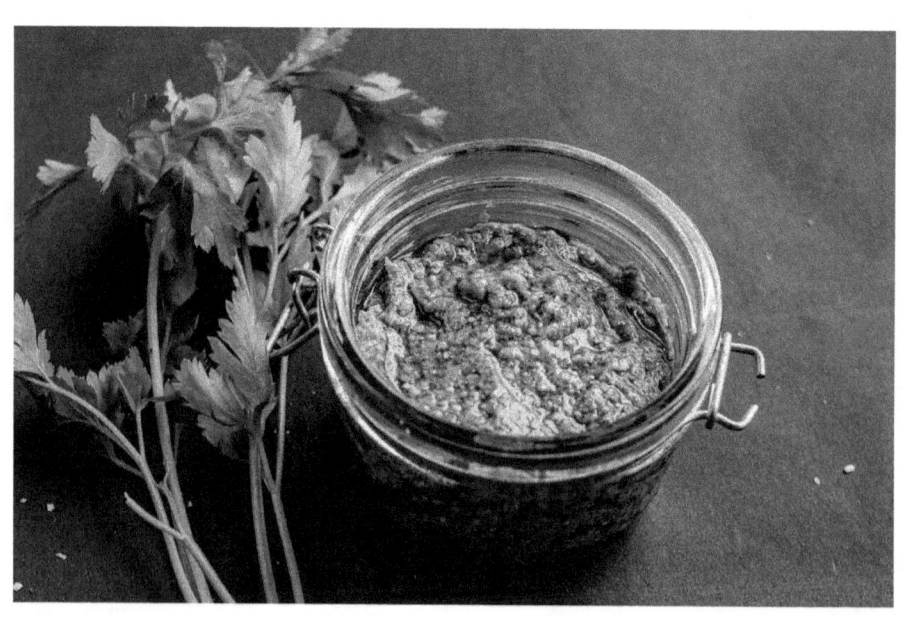

Quinoa with Pumpkin

Preparation Time: 5 minutes

Cooking Time: 20 minutes

Servings: 6

Ingredients:

½ cup pumpkin, cubed
1 tbsp. lemon juice
1 tsp. liquid honey
1 cup quinoa
2 cups of water
¼ cup of organic almond milk

Directions:

1. Put almond milk and pumpkin in the saucepan.

2. Add lemon juice and water.

3. Cook the pumpkin for 10 minutes.

4. Then add quinoa and cook the meal for 10 minutes.

5. Remove the cooked meal from the heat, add liquid honey, and stir well.

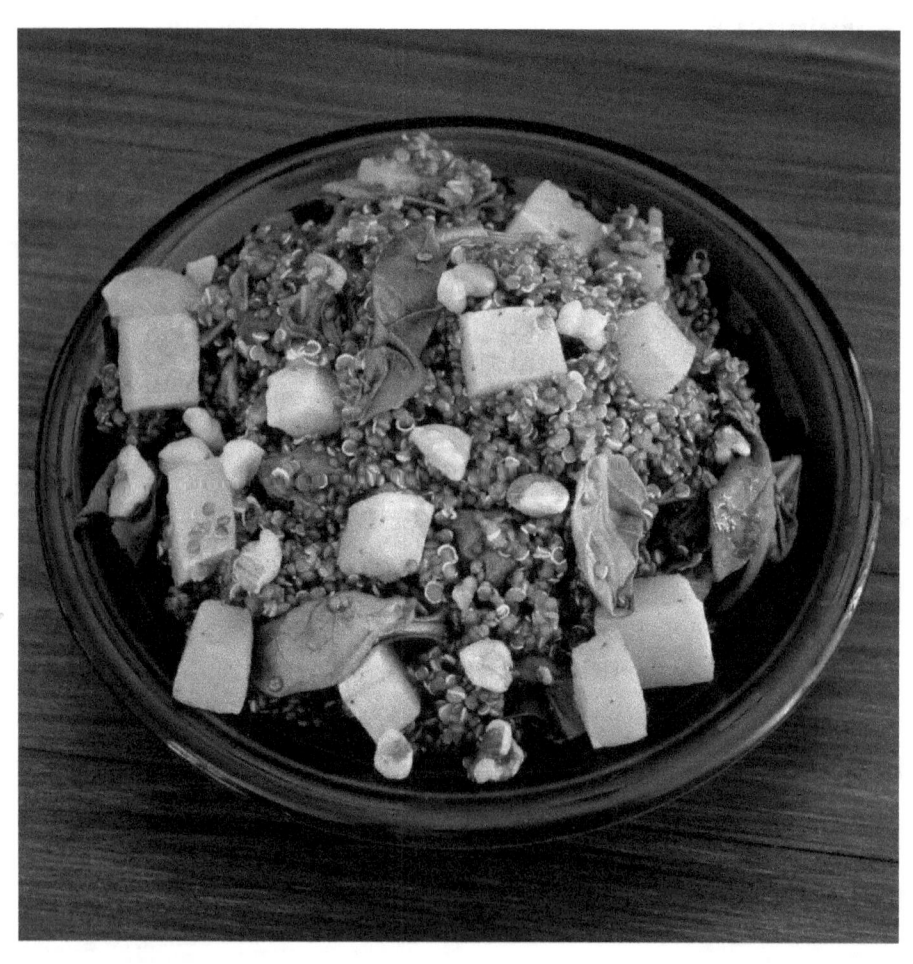

Almond Quinoa

Preparation Time: 5 minutes
Cooking Time: 4 minutes
Servings: 4

Ingredients:

1 cup quinoa
2 cups of water
1 cup organic almond milk
½ cup strawberries, sliced
1 tbsp. honey

Directions:

1. Pour water and milk in the saucepan and bring to boil.

2. Add quinoa and cook it for 12 minutes.

3. Then cool the cooked quinoa and add honey. Stir.

4. Transfer the quinoa in the bowls and top with strawberries.

Mushroom Quinoa Skillet

Preparation Time: 10 minutes

Cooking Time: 25 minutes

Servings: 6

Ingredients:
1 cup mushrooms, sliced
½ cup of water 1 tbsp. olive oil
1 tsp. Italian seasonings
½ cup quinoa
½ cup organic almond milk
¼ tsp. dried thyme

Directions:

1. Roast mushrooms with olive oil in the saucepan for 10 minutes.

2. Then stir them well, add Italian seasonings, dried thyme, and quinoa.

3. Add almond milk and water.

4. Close the lid and simmer the meal for 15 minutes. Stir it from time to time to avoid burning.

Strawberry Quinoa Bowl

Preparation Time: 15 minutes

Cooking Time: 0 minutes

Servings: 8

Ingredients:
2 ½ cup quinoa, cooked
¼ cup strawberries, roughly chopped
½ cup fresh spinach, chopped
2 pecans, chopped
1 tbsp. balsamic vinegar
1 tsp. avocado oil

Directions:

1. Mix quinoa, fresh spinach, and pecans in the big bowl.

2. Then add strawberries and avocado oil.

3. Gently shake the mixture and transfer in the serving bowls.

4. Sprinkle every serving with a small amount of balsamic vinegar.

Stir-Fried Farro

Preparation Time: 10 minutes
Cooking Time: 8minutes
Servings: 4

Ingredients:

1 cup farro, cooked
1 egg, beaten
1 tbsp. olive oil
½ tsp. chili flakes

Directions:

1. Heat olive oil and egg beaten egg.

2. Cook it for 1 minute and then stir it carefully.

3. Add cooked farro and chili flakes.

4. Fry the meal for 7 minutes. Stir it from time to time.

Quick Farro Skillet

Preparation Time: 10 minutes
Cooking Time: 15 minutes
Servings: 6

Ingredients:

2 oz fresh spinach, chopped
2 oz asparagus, chopped
1/3 cup farro, cooked
1 tbsp. olive oil
½ tsp. curry powder

Directions:

1. Line the skillet with baking paper.

2. Put all ingredients in the prepared skillet, flatten them gently and transfer in the preheated to 365°F oven.

3. Cook the meal for 15 minutes.

Bulgur Bowl

Preparation Time: 10 minutes
Cooking Time: 0 minutes
Servings: 4

Ingredients:

6 oz salmon, boiled, chopped
½ cup bulgur, cooked
1 cup fresh cilantro, chopped 1 cup tomato, chopped
3 tbsp. lemon juice 1 tbsp. olive oil

Directions:

1. Put salmon, bulgur, cilantro, and tomato in the bowl.

2. Add lemon juice and olive oil.

3. Shake the mixture well and transfer in the serving bowls.

Boiled Bulgur with Kale

Preparation Time: 10 minutes
Cooking Time: 11 minutes
Servings: 6

Ingredients:

1 cup bulgur cups water
1 cup kale
½ zucchini, chopped
½ tsp. allspices
6 tbsp. olive oil
2 oz goat cheese, crumbled

Directions:

1. Mix water and bulgur in the saucepan and cook boil for 11 minutes.

2. Then cool the bulgur and mix it with chopped kale, zucchini, allspices, and olive oil.

3. Transfer the bulgur meal in the serving bowls and top with goat cheese.

Chicken and Rice Soup

Preparation Time: 10 minutes

Cooking Time: 20 minutes

Servings: 6

Ingredients:

4 cups chicken stock 1 cup of water
1-lb. chicken breast, shredded 1 cup of rice, cooked
3 egg yolks
3 tbsp. lemon juice
1/3 cup fresh parsley, chopped
½ tsp. salt
¼ tsp. ground black pepper

Directions:

1. Pour water and chicken stock in the saucepan and bring to boil.

2. Then pour one cup of the hot liquid in the food processor.

3. Add cooked rice, egg yolks, lemon juice, and salt. Blend the mixture until smooth.

4. After this, transfer the smooth rice mixture into the saucepan with remaining chicken stock liquid.

5. Add shredded chicken breast, parsley, and ground black pepper.
6. Boil the soup for 5 minutes more.

Tomato Bulgur

Preparation Time: 5 minutes
Cooking Time: 20 minutes
Servings: 3

Ingredients:

½ cup bulgur 1 onion, diced
3 tbsp. tomato paste
½ tsp. salt
2 tbsp. olive oil 1 cup of water

Directions:

1. Melt the olive oil in the saucepan.

2. Add diced onion and cook it until light brown.

3. Then add bulgur and tomato paste. Stir the ingredients.

4. Add water and cook the meal for 15 minutes.

Well spiced Lentil Soup with sour taste

Cooking and preparation: 45 minutes
Serves: 6

Ingredients:

6 cups water –
1 diced celery stalk -
2 tbsps olive oil –
1oregano sprig -
1chopped shallot –
1thyme sprig -
1chopped garlic clove –
1/2diced tomatoes
1cored and diced green bell pepper
4sliced rhubarb stalks
5cored and diced yellow bell pepper
6green lentils
7diced carrot
8vegetable stock
9Salt and pepper to taste

Directions:

1.In a soup pot, heat the oil and stir in the garlic, bell peppers, shallots, carrot and celery.

2.Soften it by cooking for 5 minutes and add stock, the lentils, water, rhubarb and water, also add tomatoes.

3.Add oregano sprig and thyme after seasoning with pepper and salt.

4.For 20 minutes, cook on low heat.

5. Best served chilled or warm.

Delicious and entertaining Lamb Veggie Soup

Cooking and preparation: 1 ½ hour
Serves: 8

Ingredients:

6 cups water – 6 cups
½ cubed pound lamb shoulder – 1 1 2
2 tbsps lemon juice – 2 tbsps
2 cups cauliflower florets – 2 cups
2 tbsps olive oil – 2 tbsps
1 basil sprig - 1
1 chopped shallots – 2
1 crushed tomatoes – 1 can
2 diced carrots – 2
1 thyme sprig - 1
2 diced celery stalks – 2
½ cup green peas – ½ cup
¼ tsp grated ginger – ¼ tsp
4 cups vegetable stock – 4 cups
1 oregano sprig - 1
Pepper and salt to taste

Directions:

1. In a soup pot, heat the oil and stir in the lamb shoulder.

2. Add stock and water after cooking on all sides for 5 minutes.

3. Add the remaining Ingredients: after cooking for 40 minutes and season with pepper and salt.

4.Cook it for another 20 minutes and serve the soup when it's still fresh.

Bulgur Mix

Preparation Time: 10 minutes

Cooking Time: 0 minutes

Servings: 3

Ingredients:

½ cup bulgur, cooked
¼ cup corn kernels, cooked
¼ cup chickpeas, cooked
¼ cup snap peas, cooked 4 tbsp. plain yogurt

Directions:

1. Put all ingredients in the big bowl and carefully stir.

Aromatic Baked Brown Rice

Preparation Time: 10 minutes

Cooking Time: 20 minutes

Servings: 6

Ingredients:

½ cup minced fresh parsley
¾ cup jarred roasted red peppers, rinsed, patted dry, and chopped
1 cup chicken or vegetable broth
1½ cups long-grain brown rice, rinsed 2 onions, chopped fine
2¼ cups water
4 tsp. extra-virgin olive oil Grated Parmesan cheese Lemon wedges Salt and pepper

Directions:

1. Place the oven rack in the centre of the oven and pre-heat your oven to 375°F. Heat oil in a Dutch oven on moderate heat until it starts to shimmer. Put in onions and 1 tsp. salt and cook, stirring intermittently, till they become tender and well browned, 12 to 14 minutes.

2. Mix in water and broth and bring to boil. Mix in rice, cover, and move pot to oven. Bake until rice becomes soft and liquid is absorbed, 65 to 70 minutes.

3. Remove pot from oven. Sprinkle red peppers over rice, cover, and allow to sit for about five minutes. Put in parsley to rice and fluff gently with fork to combine. Sprinkle with salt and pepper to taste. Serve with grated Parmesan and lemon wedges.

Aromatic Barley Pilaf

Preparation Time: 10 minutes
Cooking Time: 10 minutes
Servings: 6

Ingredients:

¼ cup minced fresh parsley 1 small onion, chopped fine
1½ cups pearl barley, rinsed 1½ tsp. lemon juice
1½ tsp. minced fresh thyme or ½ tsp. dried 2 garlic cloves, minced
2 tbsp. minced fresh chives 2½ cups water
3 tbsp. extra-virgin olive oil Salt and pepper

Directions:

1. Heat oil in a big saucepan on moderate heat until it starts to shimmer. Put in onion and ½ tsp. salt and cook till they become tender, approximately five minutes. Mix in barley, garlic, and thyme and cook, stirring often, until barley is lightly toasted and aromatic, approximately three minutes.

2. Mix in water and bring to simmer. Decrease heat to low, cover, and simmer until barley becomes soft and water is absorbed, 20 to 40 minutes.

3. Remove from the heat, lay clean dish towel underneath lid and let pilaf sit for about ten minutes. Put in parsley, chives, and lemon juice to pilaf and fluff gently with fork to combine. Sprinkle with salt and pepper to taste. Serve.

Basmati Rice Pilaf Mix

Preparation Time: 10 minutes
Cooking Time: 15 minutes

Ingredients:

¼ cup currants
¼ cup sliced almonds, toasted
¼ tsp. ground cinnamon
½ tsp. ground turmeric
1 small onion, chopped fine
1 tbsp. extra-virgin olive oil
1½ cups basmati rice, rinsed
2 garlic cloves, minced
2¼ cups water
Salt and pepper

Directions:

1. Heat oil in a big saucepan on moderate heat until it starts to shimmer. Put in onion and ¼ tsp. salt and cook till they become tender, approximately five minutes. Put in rice, garlic, turmeric, and cinnamon and cook, stirring often, until grain edges begin to turn translucent, approximately three minutes.

2. Mix in water and bring to simmer. Decrease heat to low, cover, and simmer gently until rice becomes soft and water is absorbed, 16 to 18 minutes.

3. Remove from the heat, drizzle currants over pilaf. Cover, laying clean dish towel underneath lid, and let pilaf sit for about ten minutes. Put in almonds to pilaf and fluff gently with fork to combine. Sprinkle with salt and pepper to taste. Serve.

Brown Rice Salad with Asparagus, Goat Cheese, and Lemon

Preparation Time: 10 minutes

Cooking Time: 15 minutes

Servings: 2

Ingredients:

¼ cup minced fresh parsley
¼ cup slivered almonds, toasted
1 lb. asparagus, trimmed and cut into 1-inch lengths
1 shallot, minced
1 tsp. grated lemon zest plus
3 tbsp. juice
1½ cups long-grain brown rice
2 oz. goat cheese, crumbled (½ cup)
3½ tbsp. extra-virgin olive oil
Salt and pepper

Directions:

1. Bring 4 quarts water to boil in a Dutch oven. Put in rice and 1½ tsp. salt and cook, stirring intermittently, until rice is tender, about half an hour. Drain rice, spread onto rimmed baking sheet, and drizzle with 1 tbsp. lemon juice. Allow it to cool completely, about fifteen minutes.

2. Heat 1 tbsp. oil in 12-inch frying pan on high heat until just smoking. Put in asparagus, ¼ tsp. salt, and ¼ tsp. pepper and cook, stirring intermittently, until asparagus is browned and crisp-tender, about 4 minutes; move to plate and allow to cool slightly.

3. Beat remaining 2½ tbsp. oil, lemon zest and remaining 2 tbsp. juice, shallot, ½ tsp. salt, and ½ tsp. pepper together in a big container.

4. Put in rice, asparagus, 2 tbsp. goat cheese, 3 tbsp. almonds, and 3 tbsp. parsley. Gently toss to combine and allow to sit for about ten minutes. Sprinkle with salt and pepper to taste.

5. Move to serving platter and drizzle with remaining 2 tbsp. goat cheese, remaining 1 tbsp. almonds, and remaining 1 tbsp. parsley. Serve.

Carrot-Almond-Bulgur Salad

Preparation Time: 10 minutes

Cooking Time: 20 minutes

Servings: 4

Ingredients:

1/8 tsp. cayenne pepper
1/3 cup chopped fresh cilantro
1/3 cup chopped fresh mint
1/3 cup extra-virgin olive oil
½ cup sliced almonds, toasted
½ tsp. ground cumin 1 cup water
1½ cups medium-grind bulgur, rinsed
3 scallions, sliced thin
4 carrots, peeled and shredded
6 tbsp. lemon juice (2 lemons)
Salt and pepper

Directions:

1. Mix bulgur, water, ¼ cup lemon juice, and ¼ tsp. salt in a container. Cover and sit at room temperature until grains are softened and liquid is fully absorbed, about 1½ hours.

2. Beat remaining 2 tbsp. lemon juice, oil, cumin, cayenne, and ½ tsp. salt together in a big container.

3. Put in bulgur, carrots, scallions, almonds, mint, and cilantro and gently toss to combine. Sprinkle with salt and pepper to taste. Serve.

Chickpea-Spinach Bulgur

Preparation Time: 5 minutes

Cooking Time: 20 minutes

Servings: 6

Ingredients:

¾ cup chicken or vegetable broth
¾ cup water
1 (15-oz.) can chickpeas, rinsed
1 cup medium-grind bulgur, rinsed 1 onion, chopped fine 1 tbsp. lemon juice 2 tbsp. za'atar
3 garlic cloves, minced
3oz. (3 cups) baby spinach, chopped 3 tbsp. extra-virgin olive oil
Salt and pepper

Directions:

1. Heat 2 tbsp. oil in a big saucepan on moderate heat until it starts to shimmer. Put in onion and ½ tsp. salt and cook till they become tender, approximately five minutes. Mix in garlic and 1 tbsp. za'atar and cook until aromatic, approximately half a minute.

2. Mix in bulgur, chickpeas, broth, and water and bring to simmer. Decrease heat to low, cover, and simmer gently until bulgur is tender, 16 to 18 minutes.

3. Remove from the heat, lay clean dish towel underneath lid and let bulgur sit for about ten minutes. Put in spinach, lemon juice, remaining 1 tbsp. za'atar, and residual 1 tbsp. oil and fluff gently with fork to combine. Sprinkle with salt and pepper to taste. Serve.

Classic Baked Brown Rice

Preparation Time: 10 minutes

Cooking Time: 20 minutes

Servings: 6

Ingredients:

1½ cups long-grain brown rice, rinsed
2 tsp. extra-virgin olive oil
2 1/3 cups boiling water Salt and pepper

Directions:

1. Place the oven rack in the centre of the oven and preheat your oven to 375°F. Mix boiling water, rice, oil, and ½ tsp. salt in 8-inch square baking dish.

2. Cover dish tightly using double layer of aluminium foil. Bake until rice becomes soft and water is absorbed, about 1 hour. Remove the dish from oven, uncover, and gently fluff rice with fork, scraping up any rice stuck to the bottom.

3. Cover dish with clean dish towel and let rice sit for about five minutes. Uncover and let rice sit for about five minutes longer.

4. Sprinkle with salt and pepper to taste. Serve.

Classic Italian Seafood Risotto

Preparation Time: 10 minutes

Cooking Time: 20 minutes

Servings: 4

Ingredients:

1/8 tsp. saffron threads, crumbled
1 (14.5-oz.) can diced tomatoes, drained
1 cup dry white wine
1 onion, chopped fine 1 tbsp. lemon juice
1 tsp. minced fresh thyme or ¼ tsp. dried
12 oz. large shrimp (26 to 30 per lb.), peeled and deveined, shells reserved
 12 oz. small bay scallops 2 bay leaves
2Cups Arborio rice 2 cups chicken broth
2 tbsp. minced fresh parsley 2½ cups water
4 (8-oz.) bottles clam juice
5 garlic cloves, minced
5 tbsp. extra-virgin olive oil
Salt and pepper

Directions:

1.Bring shrimp shells, broth, water, clam juice, tomatoes, and bay leaves to boil in a big saucepan on moderate to high heat.

2.Decrease the heat to a simmer and cook for 20 minutes. Strain mixture through fine-mesh strainer into big container, pressing on solids to extract as much liquid as possible; discard solids. Return broth to now-empty saucepan, cover, and keep warm on low heat.

3. Heat 2 tbsp. oil in a Dutch oven on moderate heat until it starts to shimmer. Put in onion and cook till they become tender, approximately five minutes.

4. Put in rice, garlic, thyme, and saffron and cook, stirring often, until grain edges begin to turn translucent, approximately three minutes.

5. Put in wine and cook, stirring often, until fully absorbed, approximately three minutes. Mix in 3½ cups warm broth, bring to simmer, and cook, stirring intermittently, until almost fully absorbed, about fifteen minutes.

6 Carry on cooking rice, stirring often and adding warm broth, 1 cup at a time, every few minutes as liquid is absorbed, until rice is creamy and cooked through but still somewhat firm in center, about fifteen minutes.

7 Mix in shrimp and scallops and cook, stirring often, until opaque throughout, approximately three minutes. Remove pot from heat, cover, and allow to sit for about five minutes.

8. Adjust consistency with remaining warm broth as required (you may have broth left over). Mix in remaining 3 tbsp. oil, parsley, and lemon juice and sprinkle with salt and pepper to taste. Serve.

Classic Stovetop White Rice

Preparation Time: 10 minutes

Cooking Time: 10 minutes

Servings: 6

Ingredients:

1 tbsp. extra-virgin olive oil
2 cups long-grain white rice, rinsed
3 cups water
long-grain rice can substitute basmati, jasmine, or Texmati rice for the long-grain rice.
Salt and pepper

Directions:

1.Heat oil in a big saucepan on moderate heat until it starts to shimmer. Put in rice and cook, stirring frequently, until grain edges begin to turn translucent, approximately two minutes.

2.Put in water and 1 tsp. salt and bring to simmer. Cover, decrease the heat to low, and simmer gently until rice becomes soft and water is absorbed, approximately twenty minutes.

3.Remove from the heat, lay clean dish towel underneath lid and let rice sit for about ten minutes. Gently fluff rice with fork. Sprinkle with salt and pepper to taste. Serve.

Chicken Sausage Minestrone

Preparation time: 10 minutes

Cooking time :30 minutes

Servings:4

Ingredients:

4 sliced chicken sausage
4 tomatoes; sliced and peeled
2 chopped cloves
½ pound of diced green beans
2 sliced carrots
A dubbed zucchini
2 tbsps Olive oil;
1 diced sweet onion
½ cup of green peas; frozen
1 sliced celery stalk
2 cups of vegetable stalk
½ cup of marjoram; dried
6 cups Water;
½ teaspoon of oregano; dried
½ teaspoon of basil; dried
Pepper and salt to taste

Directions:

1.Get a soup pot and heat the oil, then pour in your chicken sausage and some diced onion, then cook for 5 minutes.

2.Now, add in your tomatoes, carrot, cloves, onion and celery and wait till it's cooked for another 10 minutes then add your remaining Ingredients:.

3.Add pepper and salt to taste, then cook for 20 minutes.

4.Serve and enjoy your soup when warm.

Italian Lentil soup

Preparation time: 15 minutes

Cooking time: 30 minutes

Servings: 6

Ingredients:

2 tbsp of sliced parsley
2 tbsp Tomato paste;
2 tbsp Olive Oil;
2 sliced cloves
1 cup of sliced tomatoes
2 celery stalks; chopped
2 sliced shallots
2 carrots; chopped
¼ cup of red wine
6 cups Water; 6 cups
A basil sprig
A thyme sprigs
An oregano sprig
1 cup Green lentils; 1 cup
2 cups of vegetable stock
Pepper and salt to taste

Directions:

1.Get a soup pot and heat your olive oil, then pour in your chopped celery, clove, carrots and shallot, then cook for 5 minutes before adding your vegetable stock, lentils, tomatoes, wine and water.

2.Join in the herbs, then add pepper and salt to taste and then cook for 25 minutes.

3.After 25 minutes, add your sliced parsley in and serve your warm soup.

Smoked chicken sausage soup

Preparation time: 10 minutes

Cooking time: 30 minutes

Servings: 4

Ingredients:

2 sliced chicken sausage
2 sliced smoked chicken sausage
1 can of sliced tomatoes
1 onion, sliced
2 cups Water; 2 cups
2 cups Vegetable stock; 2 cups
1 celery stalk; chopped
2 tbsp Chopped cilantro; 2 tablespoons
2 tbsp Olive Oil; 2 tablespoons
Pepper and salt to taste

Directions:

1. Get a soup pot and heat your olive oil, then pour in your sausage and cook for 5 minutes. After that, pour in your sliced onion, tomatoes, celery and carrots and cook for another 5 minutes.

2. Now, add your short pasta and water with pepper and salt to taste, then cook for 20 minutes.

3. After 20 minutes, pour in your chopped parsley and cilantro then serve after cooling.

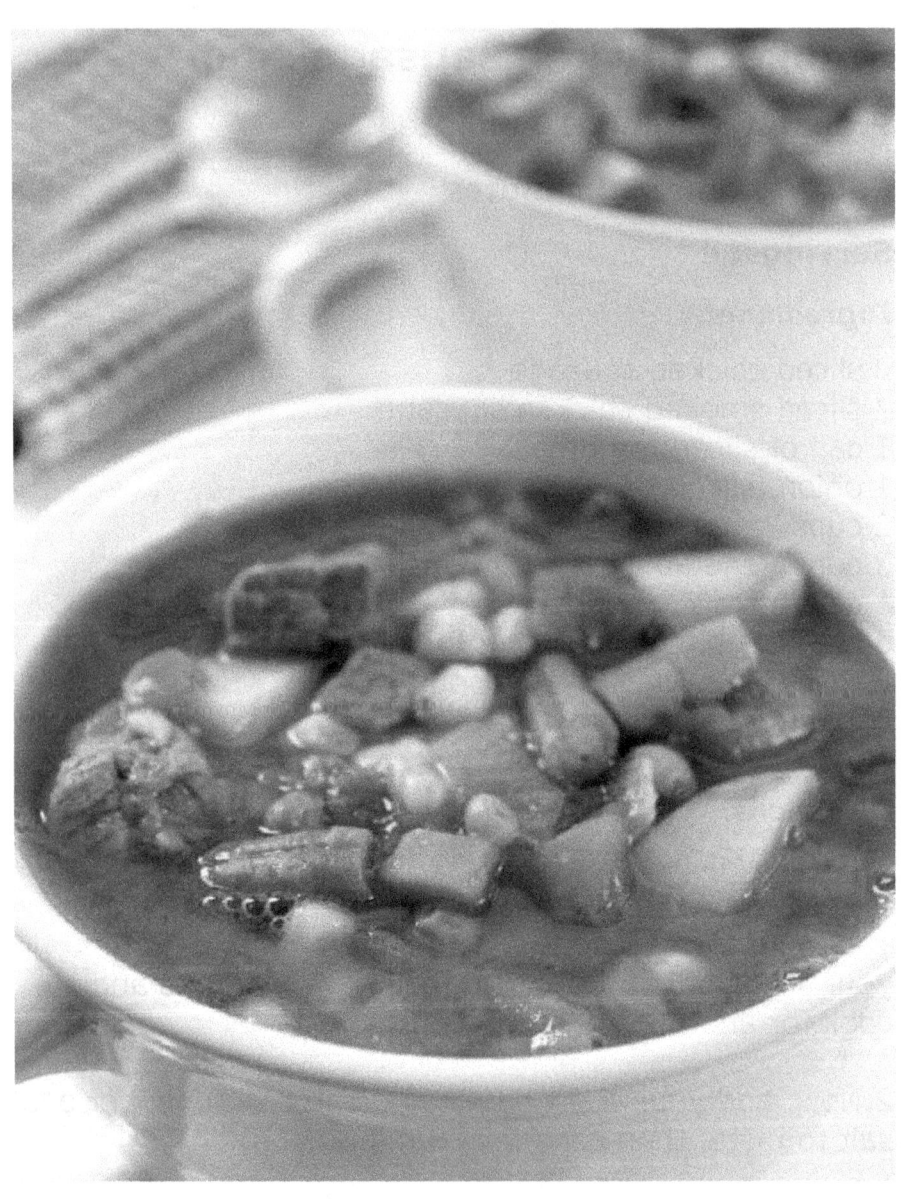

Lemon Chicken Soup

Preparation Time: 10 minutes

Cooking Time: 20 minutes

Servings: 6

Ingredients:

10 cups chicken broth 3 tbsp. olive oil
8 cloves garlic, minced 1 sweet onion, sliced
1 large lemon, zested
2 boneless skinless chicken breasts 1 cup Israeli couscous
1/2 tsp. crushed red pepper 2 oz. crumbled feta
1/3 cup chopped chive Salt and pepper, to taste

Directions:

1. Grab a stock pot, add the oil and place over a medium heat.

2. Add the onion and garlic and cook for five minutes until soft.

3. Add the broth, chicken breasts, lemon zest and crushed pepper.

4. Raise the heat, cover and bring to a boil.

5 Reduce the heat then simmer for 5 minutes.

6. Turn off the heat, remove the lid and remove the chicken from the pot.

7.Pop onto a place and use two forks to shred.
8Pop back into the pot, add the feta, chives and salt and pepper.

9Stir well then serve and enjoy.

Tuscan Vegetable Pasta Soup

Preparation Time: 10 minutes

Cooking Time: 30 minutes

Servings: 6

Ingredients:

2 tbsp. extra virgin olive oil 4 cloves garlic, minced
1 medium yellow onion, diced 1/2 cup carrot, chopped
1/2 cup celery, chopped
1 medium zucchini, sliced and quartered 1 x 15 oz. can diced tomatoes
6 cups vegetable stock 2 tbsp. tomato paste
6-8 oz. whole wheat pasta 1 x 15 oz. can white beans
2 large handfuls baby spinach 6 basil cubes
Salt and pepper, to taste
Fresh chopped parsley, for garnish

Directions:
1. Grab a stock pot, add the oil and pop over a medium heat.
2. Add the onion and garlic and cook for five minutes until soft.

3. Throw in the carrots, celery and zucchini and cook for an extra 5 minutes, stirring occasionally.

4. Add the tomato and salt and pepper and cook for 1-2 minutes.

5. Add the veggies broth and tomato paste, stir well then bring to the boil.

6.Throw in the pasta, cook for 10 minutes then add the spinach, white beans, basil cubes and seasoning.

7Stir well then remove from the heat.

8.Divide between large bowls and serve and enjoy.

Dairy Free Zucchini Soup

Preparation Time: 10 minutes

Cooking Time: 25 minutes

Servings: 8

Ingredients:

2½ lb. zucchini
1 medium onion, diced
2 tbsp. olive oil
4 garlic cloves, chopped
4 cups chicken stock
Sea salt and pepper, to taste
1/3 cup fresh basil leaves

Directions:

1. Grab a pan, add the oil and pop over a medium heat.

2. Add the onion, garlic and zucchini and cook for five minutes until soft.

3. Add the stock and simmer for 15 minutes.
Remove from the heat, stir through the basil, add the seasoning and use an immersion blender to whizz until smooth.

4. Serve and enjoy.

Farro Stew with Kale & Cannellini Beans

Preparation Time: 10 minutes

Cooking Time 1 hour

Servings: 4

Ingredients:

2 tbsp. olive oil
2 medium carrots, diced
1 medium onion, chopped
2 sticks celery, chopped
4 cloves garlic, minced
5 cups low-sodium vegetable broth
1 x 14.5 oz. can diced tomatoes
1 cup farro, rinsed
1 tsp. dried oregano
1 bay leaf
Salt, to taste
1/2 cup parsley
4 cups chopped kale, thick ribs removed
1 x 15 oz. can cannellini beans, drained and rinsed
1 tbsp. fresh lemon juice
1/2 cup feta cheese, crumbled

Directions:

1.Grab a stock pot, add the oil and place over a medium heat.

2Add the onion, carrots and celery and cook for five minutes until becoming soft.

3.Add the garlic and cook for another 30 seconds.

4.Stir through the broth, tomatoes, farro, oregano, bay leaf, parsley and salt.

5.Cover with the lid and bring to the boil. Reduce the heat then simmer for 20 minutes.

6.Remove the lid, add the kale and cook for a further 10-15 minutes.

7.Remove the bay leaf, add the beans, stir through the lemon juice and any additional liquid then stir well to combine.
Serve and enjoy

www.ingramcontent.com/pod-product-compliance
Lightning Source LLC
Chambersburg PA
CBHW070722030426
42336CB00013B/1892